LITTLE BOOK OF

NAIL
TIPS

LINDA BUTTLE

GW00706192

LITTLE BOOK OF
NAIL
TIPS

LINDA BUTTLE

Ruby
BOOKS

Ruby Books
Scarborough House
29 James Street West
Bath BA1 2BT

Phone 44 (0) 1225 316013 **Fax** 44 (0) 1225 445836
E-mail rubybooks@absolutepress.co.uk
Web www.absolutepress.co.uk

Written by Linda Buttle
The author has asserted her moral rights.

Designed by Blue Sunflower Creative
Series Editor Meg Avent

A catalogue record of this book is available
from the British Library

ISBN 0 954987 10 1

Printed and bound by Legoprint, Italy

50 fabulous tips on

how to achieve beautiful nails.

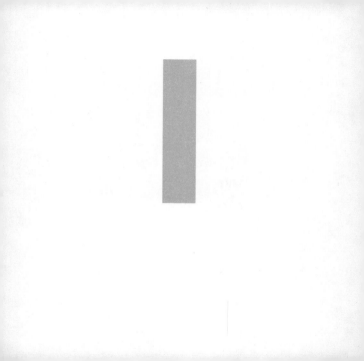

Have a professional manicurist **analyse your nails;** that way you'll be able to get the best advice on the **right products** to use **for your nail type.**

2

Keep **hand and cuticle cream** somewhere obvious, such as on your desk or by your bed; this will help you remember to **apply it regularly.**

3

Try **exfoliating the backs of your hands** with a face or body scrub. Used once a week your hands will be kept feeling silky smooth.

If you've **chipped a nail** you don't have to completely redo your manicure. Instead, ask somebody else to apply remover to just that one nail so you **don't risk spoiling the rest.**

5

Carry nail plasters in your handbag so that if you catch a nail you can keep it in place until you can do a proper repair job.

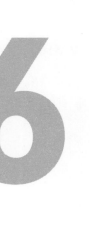

Aim to balance your 'look', so
if you've got high shine or
shimmery nails
opt for **matt make-up**
or vice versa.

Rest your hands on a firm surface, such as a tabletop, to give you a steady hand **when applying polish.**

8

Do like the professionals do and always apply a **base and topcoat** when painting your nails. You'll find it really helps to **lengthen the life of your nail polish.**

For a **long lasting effect** it pays to remember that **two thin layers of polish** are far better than one thick one.

10

If your hands are prone to dryness,

treat yourself to a salon

paraffin wax or hot oil mitt treatment to boost the

condition of both your hands and nails.

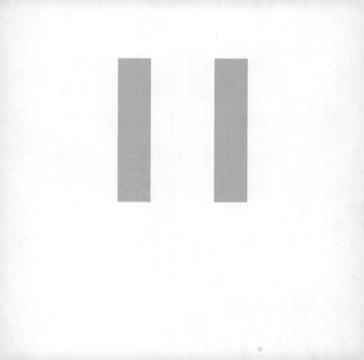

Apply the first stroke of polish down the middle of the nail and then a stroke either side to **prevent clogging around the cuticles.**

12

Smooth out ridges

on your nails with regular buffing and

use a ridge-filling basecoat for a perfect polish finish.

13

For **touch-dry nails in next to no time** use a fast-drying spray once you've finished your manicure. Alternatively, use your hairdryer to blow warm air to help set your polish.

Rubbing cuticle oil into your toe nails

and then soaking them in

warm water will
soften the nails

and make them easier to cut.

15

For a **homemade hand and nail scrub:** mix one teaspoon of olive oil with one tablespoon of sugar and massage it in for a minute. Rinse with warm water and **feel that smoothness!**

16

Sand makes a great exfoliator. Taking a long walk along the beach will leave your feet feeling smooth and your nails shining.

Dehydration is a major cause of **dry, brittle and flaking nails,** so be sure to **drink plenty of water.**

18

To get rid of unsightly cuticles rub in a cuticle remover, then, after a couple of minutes, push them back gently with an orange stick. Never be tempted to cut your cuticles, this is a job best left to a professional.

19

Keep **nail polish** in **the refrigerator** to prevent it from thickening in the bottle.

20

For a neat finish to your manicure, dip a cotton wool bud or small brush in nail varnish remover to clean up the edges, or buy a specialist corrector pen.

21

Always apply a clear **basecoat;**

it acts as a barrier and

prevents staining of the nail.

22

If your **nails have become stained,** apply a little **lemon juice and buff** with a nailbrush to whiten them.

23

Nails don't have to be long to look well groomed. In fact **bright colours** can often look **over the top on long nails.**

24

Nail varnish remover

can be very drying so always opt for

one with an **oil-based**

conditioning formula

without any acetone.

25

Cut toe nails straight across rather than in a curve which encourages in-growing toe nails. Any sharp edges can then be filed with the coarse side of an emery board.

26

Protect your hands and nails by always wearing **gloves for washing-up** and other household chores. Gloves also prevent you from being tempted to use your nails as tools, which is a sure-fire way to damage them.

27

Take some flip-flops

or open-toed sandals with you

when you have a professional pedicure,

as the polish may feel dry to the touch

but will actually take a good hour to

fully harden.

28

Use a fine-grade emery board and **file in just one direction** rather than using a sawing action, which can easily damage the nail.

29

If you have problems achieving your

own French manicure, use a white nail pencil

to whiten the nail tips rather than

polish. You'll find it much easier

to work with.

30

'Barely there' **pastel shades** are ideal **for hard-working hands,** as chips are far less likely to show up than with deeper shades.

31

Handy **travel-size packets** of individually wrapped wipes soaked in **nail varnish remover** are ideal to take with you on your travels.

32

Don't look old before your time by neglecting your hands: always use a **hand cream with an SPF** or apply sunscreen to the backs of your hands during the summer.

33

If you file and **reshape your nails every week** they will not only be kept in great shape, but they will also be less likely to split.

34

At the start of your manicure, apply a little nail varnish remover, even if you don't have any colour on your nails. This will **help the polish to grip your nail** better and prolong the life of your manicure.

35

If you suffer with very soft nails, try **filing** them **while you're still wearing nail polish.**

You'll find it helps to prevent cracking.

36

To **prevent bubbles** appearing **in your polish,** don't shake the bottle before applying it; simply roll it around in your hands.

37

If you break a nail be sure to trim all your nails to the same length. **Nothing looks worse** than **odd length nails.**

38

Never use **metal nail** files: they are far **too harsh** and do more harm than good.

39

Hangnails are best **removed** by using **specialist scissors.** Prevention, though, is always better than cure and you can do this by massaging in cuticle oil on a daily basis.

40

If you're **not brave enough to wear bright colours** on your hands, **try them out on your toes** first and see how you feel.

White spots can be caused by a lack of vitamins and minerals, but if you've got a healthy diet they are probably just **due to a knock damaging the nail** and will soon grow out.

42

Massage your cuticles

regularly; it's a great way to

boost circulation

and improve their condition. There are

plenty of specialist nail oils you can

use but olive oil is cheaper and

just as effective.

43

Get out of the habit of nail biting by wearing artificial nails you can't bite. Alternatively, wear a bright polish that will act like a warning signal every time you're tempted to bite them.

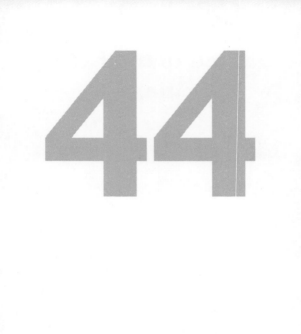

Use **toe spacers** to make applying polish much easier. Keep the toes apart and **prevent smudging.**

45

Want **high shine** without the hassle of re-applying nail varnish? **Get yourself a nail buffer,** the natural way to high shine nails.

46

Soaking your feet in a

specialist foot soak

is not only relaxing but can also

help your body to detox.

Wrap your hands and feet in food-wrap over a moisturising mask to get them to feel really soft. Or wear **cotton gloves and socks to bed** occasionally after applying a rich moisturiser.

48

Specialist **nail care supplements** taken regularly will help your **nails grow stronger** and stay supple.

49

Be ready to party! Turn daytime nails into something special; **add a coat of clear sparkly polish** over the top.

50

To **make a professional manicure last longer** take your **own polish** along **with you,** or purchase your chosen one from the salon. Any chips can then be touched up later.

Linda Buttle

Linda Buttle is a freelance
Photojournalist who specialises in
writing health, beauty and travel features
for a variety of magazines and websites.

**Second title in the
Ruby Books Beauty Series.
Published 2005:**

LITTLE BOOK OF
HAIR TIPS

No more bad hair days! From the secrets to

extra shine to how to get super-sexy curls

without the frizz. These brilliant tips are the key

to truly luscious locks.

ISBN 0 9549871 1 X